Workouts for seniors over 60

Workout to boost strength, balance, mobility, achieve weight loss and wellness also to overcome osteoporosis aging, with videos

Kevin D. Page

This book is a work of non-fiction the views expressed are solely those of the author and do not necessarily reflect the views of the publisher, and the publisher hereby disclaims any responsibility for them.

Table Of Content

Introduction

Notice: Stick to the last page for bonus videos.

This a comprehensive guide designed to help you embrace your golden years with strength, vitality, and grace. This book is not just about physical exercise, it's about empowering you to take charge of your health and well-being, no matter what your age.

As we grow older, our bodies experience a multitude of

transformations. Our muscles weaken, our bones become more fragile, and our joints start to ache.

But this doesn't mean that we have to resign ourselves to a life of inactivity and decline. On the contrary, staying active and maintaining a regular exercise routine can help us age more gracefully, prevent many age-related diseases, and even reverse some of the effects of aging.

We will explore a variety of workouts that are specifically tailored to the needs of seniors over 60. We'll cover everything from low-impact exercises that are easy on the joints, to strength training that can help you maintain or even increase your muscle mass.

We'll also delve into the importance of flexibility and balance training, as well as cardiovascular exercise to keep your heart healthy and strong.

But "Workouts for Seniors over 60" is about more than just physical fitness. It's also about mental health, social connection, and the overall quality of life. We'll discuss the many benefits of exercise for seniors, including improved mood, better sleep, and increased energy levels. We'll also provide tips and strategies for staying motivated, overcoming obstacles, and making exercise a lifelong habit.

Throughout this book, you'll find inspiring stories from other seniors who have embraced an active lifestyle and reaped the rewards. You'll also find practical advice from experts in the fields of geriatrics, fitness, and nutrition.

So, whether you're a seasoned exerciser looking for new challenges, or a beginner just starting on your fitness journey, "Workouts for Seniors over 60" is here to support you every step of the way.

Here's a real life story about a man name Liam and how he got to embrace workout into his life.

Liam, a senior over 60, had been living a sedentary lifestyle for years. His days were filled with long hours in front of the television and an unhealthy diet. He was overweight, and out of shape, and his health was deteriorating.

One day, Liam woke up with a sharp pain in his chest. He was rushed to the hospital, where doctors diagnosed him with high blood pressure and warned him about the risks of heart disease.

This was a wake-up call for Liam. He knew he needed to make changes in his life if he wanted to live longer and healthier. He decided to start working out. At first, it was difficult. His body ached, and he felt exhausted after just a few minutes of exercise.

But Liam was determined. He pushed through the pain and

discomfort, knowing that each workout brought him one step closer to better health.

Liam began by walking around his neighborhood every morning. As he walked, he noticed the beauty of nature around him - the birds chirping, the trees swaying in the breeze, and the sun rising over the horizon. These small moments of joy motivated him to keep going.

After a few weeks of walking, Liam felt stronger and more

energetic. He decided to add some strength training to his routine. He joined a local gym and started lifting weights. The gym was intimidating at first, but the other members were friendly and supportive. They helped Liam learn proper form and technique, and before long, he was making progress.

As Liam's strength increased, so did his confidence. He started to feel better about himself and his appearance. His clothes fit looser, and he noticed that he could walk upstairs without getting winded. He also began to eat healthier, swapping out junk food for fruits, vegetables, and lean proteins.

Liam's newfound health and fitness had a positive impact on his social life as well. He made friends at the gym and started attending group fitness classes. He even joined a hiking club, where he explored the great outdoors with like-minded individuals.

If Liam hadn't embraced workouts in his life he might have ended probably with worse body conditions which would have resulted in his death.

The Importance of Exercise for Seniors

Exercise is crucial for seniors as it provides numerous benefits for their physical and mental well-being. Regular physical activity can help seniors maintain their independence, mobility, and overall quality of life. Here are some specific reasons why exercise is important for seniors:

1. Physical health: Regular exercise helps seniors maintain a healthy weight, build muscle strength, improve balance, and increase flexibility. It also helps reduce the risk of chronic diseases such as heart disease, diabetes, and certain types of cancer. Engaging in physical activity also enhances cardiovascular health and strengthens the immune system.

2. Cognitive function: Exercise has been shown to improve cognitive function and reduce the risk of cognitive decline in seniors. It stimulates the brain and promotes the production of chemicals that enhance memory and learning. Regular exercise can also reduce the risk of developing Alzheimer's disease and other forms of dementia.

3. Mental health: Physical activity has a positive impact on mental well-being. Regular exercise releases endorphins, also known as "feel-good" chemicals, which boost mood and reduce symptoms of depression and anxiety. Exercise provides a sense of accomplishment and can improve self-esteem and confidence.

4. Social interaction: Participating in group exercise classes or outdoor activities provides opportunities for seniors to socialize and build relationships. Regular social interaction is vital for mental well-being and can combat feelings of loneliness and isolation, which are common among seniors.

5. Falls prevention: Exercise programs that focus on strength training, balance exercises, and flexibility can help reduce the risk of falls in seniors. Falls are a significant concern for older adults and can lead to serious injuries and a loss of independence.

6. Bone health: Weight-bearing exercises, such as walking or dancing, can help improve bone density and reduce the risk of osteoporosis and fractures in seniors.

7. Sleep quality: Regular exercise can improve the quality of sleep in seniors. Physical activity helps regulate sleep patterns and promotes a more restful and rejuvenating sleep.

Seniors need to consult with their healthcare provider before starting any exercise program to ensure their safety and identify the types and intensity of exercises suitable for their abilities and health conditions.

Overall, exercise is essential for seniors to maintain their overall health and well-being, and it should be incorporated into their daily routine.

Benefits of Regular Physical Activity Safety Considerations and Precautions

Benefits:

1.   Cardiovascular   Health: Improves heart function, reduces blood pressure, and increases circulation.

2. Weight Management: Helps maintain a healthy weight, reduces body fat, and increases muscle mass.

3. Mental Health: Reduces stress, anxiety, and depression, while improving mood and overall well-being.

4. Bone Density: Increases bone strength, reducing the risk of osteoporosis and fractures.

5. Cognitive Function: Improves concentration, memory, and problem-solving skills.

6. Sleep Quality: Enhances sleep duration and quality.

7. Immune System: Boosts immune function, reducing the risk of illness and infection.

8. Reduced Risk of Chronic Diseases: Lowers the risk of developing type 2 diabetes, certain cancers, and stroke.

Precautions and Considerations to follow

1. Consult a Doctor: Before starting a new exercise program, especially if you have any underlying medical conditions or concerns.

2. Warm-up and Cool-down: Gradually increase and decrease intensity to prevent injury and promote recovery.

3. Proper Equipment and Gear: Use appropriate gear and equipment to reduce the risk of injury.

4. Hydration: Drink plenty of water before, during, and after physical activity.

5. Listen to Your Body: Rest when needed, and stop if you experience pain or discomfort.

6. Start Slowly: Gradually increase intensity and duration to allow your body to adapt.

7. Find a Workout Buddy: Exercise with a partner or group for motivation and support.

8. Be Mindful of Your Environment: Exercise in a safe

and controlled environment, free from distractions and hazards.

Remember to prioritize your safety and well-being while enjoying the benefits of regular physical activity.

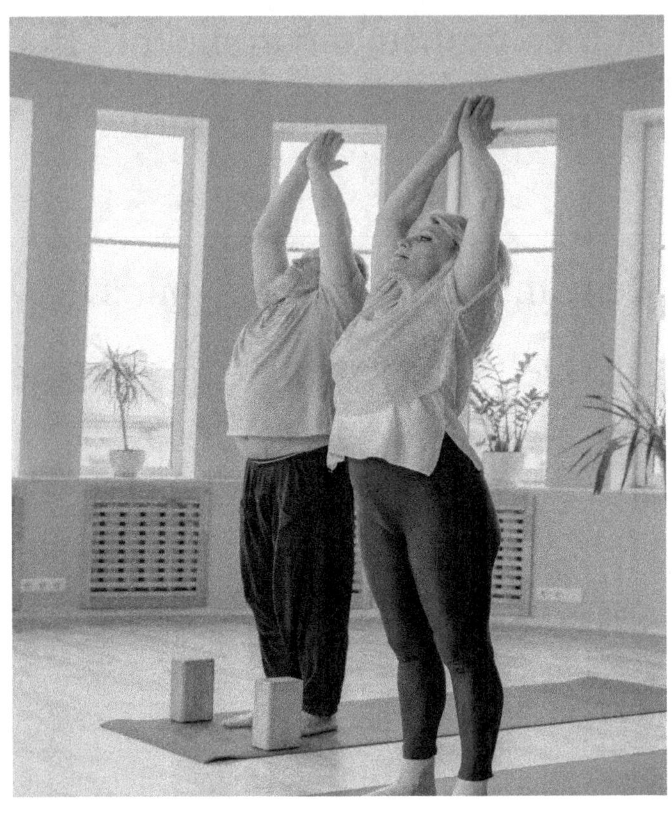

Chapter 1

Understanding Senior's Fitness Levels

Understanding senior's fitness levels is crucial to promote healthy aging and prevent age-related declines. Here are some key aspects to consider:

1. Physical Health Benefits: Regular exercise helps maintain a healthy weight, reduces the impact of illness and chronic disease, and enhances mobility, flexibility, and balance.

2. Mental Health Benefits: Exercise can improve sleep quality, boost mood and self-confidence, and improve brain function.

3. Four Building Blocks of Fitness: A balanced exercise plan should include:

- **Balance:** Exercises like yoga, tai chi, and posture exercises improve balance and reduce the risk of falls.

- **Cardio:** Activities like walking, swimming, cycling, and dancing to improve endurance and reduce fatigue.

- **Strength and Power Training:** Weightlifting, resistance band exercises, or bodyweight exercises to build muscle and improve bone density.

- **Flexibility:** Stretching exercises to improve range of motion and reduce stiffness.

Activities Beneficial to Older Adults:

- **Walking:** A low-impact exercise that requires minimal equipment.

- **Senior Sports or Fitness Classes:** Exercising with others can help with motivation and socialization.

- **Water Aerobics and Water Sports:** Low-impact exercises that reduce stress on joints.

- **Yoga:** Combines physical postures, breathing

techniques, and meditation to improve strength, flexibility, and balance.

Getting Started Safely:

- **Get Medical Clearance:** Consult with a doctor before starting a new exercise program.

- **Start Slow and Build Up Steadily:** Gradually increase exercise intensity and duration to avoid injury.

- **Listen to Your Body:** Rest when needed, and stop if

experiencing pain or discomfort.

Tips for Staying Motivated:

- **Focus on Short-term Goals:** Set achievable goals like improving mood and energy levels.

- **Reward Yourself:** Treat yourself after reaching a fitness goal or completing a workout.

- **Keep a Log:** Track progress to stay accountable and motivated.

- **Find Support:** Exercise with a friend, or family member, or join a fitness class.

Assessing Physical Fitness

Assessing physical fitness involves evaluating an individual's overall physical abilities and health status through various tests and measurements. The goals of the assessment include:

1. Recognizing one's strong points and areas of improvement

2. Setting realized goals and benchmarks

3. Developing personalized exercise programs

4. Monitoring progress and improvements

5. Identifying potential health

Common assessments include:

1. Cardiovascular endurance: Measuring heart rate, blood pressure, and oxygen consumption during exercise.

2. Muscular strength and endurance: Evaluating muscle

function through tests like push-ups, squats, and lunges.

3. Flexibility and mobility: Assessing range of motion, joint mobility, and muscle flexibility.

4. Body composition: Measuring body fat percentage, weight, and body mass index (BMI).

5. Balance and coordination: Evaluating balance, agility, and reaction time.

6. Aerobic capacity: Measuring oxygen consumption during exercise (VO2max).

7. Muscular power: Evaluating explosive strength through tests like jump squats and box jumps.

8. Functional movements: Assessing the ability to perform daily activities like walking, climbing stairs, and lifting.

Assessment tools and methods include:

1. Fitness tests: Standardized tests like the Cooper Test, Beep Test, and Sit-and-Reach Test.

2. Anthropometric measurements: Body

measurements like height, weight, and girth.

3. Physiological measurements: Heart rate, blood pressure, and oxygen saturation.

4. Questionnaires and surveys: Self-reported information on physical activity, diet, and overall health.

5. Movement screens and assessments: Evaluating movement patterns, posture, and biomechanics.

By assessing physical fitness, individuals can gain a comprehensive understanding of their physical abilities and develop targeted strategies for improvement, leading to enhanced overall health and well-being.

Common Age-Related Challenges

As people age, their bodies undergo natural changes that can impact their ability to exercise and maintain physical fitness. Here are some common age-related challenges that seniors over 60 may face when it comes to working out:

1. Decreased Muscle Mass and Strength: Loss of muscle mass and strength (sarcopenia) can make it harder to perform daily tasks and exercises.

2. Reduced Flexibility and Mobility: Stiffness and reduced range of motion can limit exercise options and increase the risk of injury.

3. Decreased Cardiovascular Endurance: Reduced heart function and lung capacity can make aerobic exercise more challenging.

4. Balance and Coordination Issues: Age-related decline in balance and coordination can increase the risk of falls and injuries.

5. Chronic Health Conditions: Managing conditions like diabetes, hypertension, arthritis, and heart disease can impact exercise choices and intensity.

6. Medication Interactions: Certain medications can interact with exercise or have side effects that impact physical performance.

7. Sleep Disturbances: Age-related sleep changes can impact recovery and exercise performance.

8. Cognitive Decline: Memory loss, confusion, or difficulty with concentration can make it harder to learn new exercises or follow instructions.

9. Social Isolation: Decreased social interaction can lead to decreased motivation and accountability.

10. Fear of Injury or Falling: Safety concerns can hold seniors back from exercising or trying new activities.

11. Decreased Bone Density: Osteoporosis can increase the risk of fractures and impact exercise choices.

12. Sensory Impairments: Vision, hearing, or sensory losses can impact exercise participation and safety.

It's essential to address these challenges with:

- Consultation with a healthcare professional or fitness expert
- Gentle progression and modification of exercises
- Incorporating exercises that improve balance, flexibility, and strength
- Using assistive devices or support when needed
- Finding social support and exercise buddies
- Focusing on functional movements and daily activities

- Celebrating small successes and progress

Chapter 2

Warm-up and Stretching Exercises

Warm-up and stretching exercises are essential for seniors to prepare their muscles for physical activity, improve flexibility, and reduce the risk of injury. Here are some gentle and effective warm-up and stretching exercises suitable for seniors:

Warm-up Exercises (5-10 minutes)

1. Light Cardio: Walking, marching in place, or jogging in place

2. Arm Circles: Hold arms straight out to the sides and make small circles

3. Leg Swings: Stand with feet hip-width apart and swing one leg forward and backward, then switch to the other leg.

4. Hip Openers: Stand with feet together and take small steps to the side, keeping the knees straight.

5. Neck Stretch: Slowly tilt the head to the side, bringing the ear towards the shoulder

Stretching Exercises (10-15 minutes)

1. Neck Stretch: Slowly tilt the head to the side, bringing the ear towards the shoulder. Hold for 30 seconds and repeat on the other side.

2. Shoulder Rolls: Roll shoulders forward and backward in a circular motion. Continue for 30 seconds.

3. Chest Stretch: Stand in a doorway with arms extended overhead and hands on the doorframe. Lean forward until a stretch is felt in the chest.Please maintain this position for a duration of 30 seconds.

4. Quad Stretch: Stand with one hand against a wall for balance and lift one leg behind, keeping the knee straight. Wait for 30 seconds and then do the same thing on the opposite side.

5. Calf Stretch: Stand with feet hip-width apart and lean forward, bending at the waist. Maintain this position for 30 seconds.

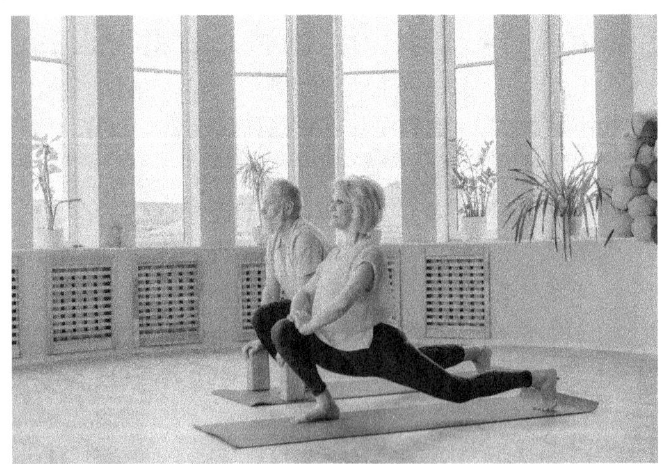

6. Hamstring Stretch: Sit on the floor with legs straight out in front. Lean forward, reaching for the toes. Maintain this position for 30 seconds.

7. Hip Flexor Stretch: Kneel on all fours. Bring one knee forward and place the foot flat on the ground in front of the other knee. Lean forward, stretching the hip flexor. Hold for 30 seconds and repeat on the other side.

8. Lower Back Stretch: Stand with feet hip-width apart and interlace fingers behind the back. Lean back, stretching the lower back. Maintain this position for 30 seconds.

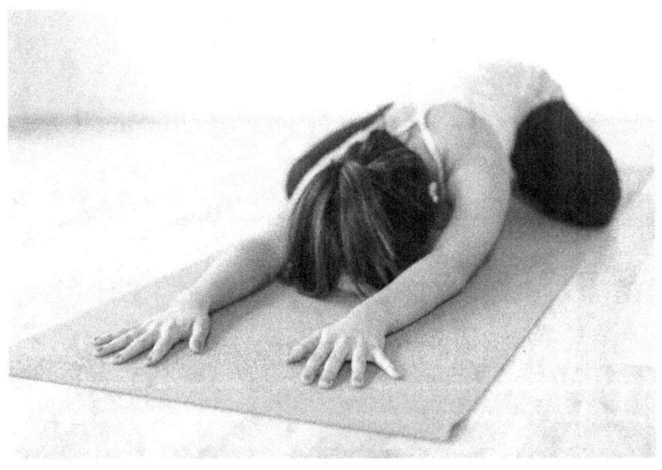

Remember to:

- Breathe naturally and smoothly while stretching.

- Don't bounce or force beyond a comfortable range.

- Hold each stretch for 30 seconds to allow for maximum relaxation of the muscles.

- Stretch after exercise or at the end of the day to improve flexibility and reduce muscle soreness.

Consult with a healthcare professional or fitness expert to

modify or add exercises based on individual needs and abilities.

Importance of Warm-up

Warm-up workouts are crucial for seniors over 60 as they prepare the body for physical activity, reduce the risk of injury, and improve overall performance. Here are the importance of warm-up workouts for seniors over 60:

1. Injury Prevention: Warm-ups reduce the risk of muscle strains, pulls, and tears by increasing blood flow and temperature in the muscles.

2. Improved Flexibility: Warm-ups increase flexibility and range of motion, making it easier to move and perform daily activities.

3. Cardiovascular Health: Warm-ups get the heart rate up and blood flowing, preparing the cardiovascular system for physical activity.

4. Reduced Muscle Soreness: Warm-ups can reduce muscle soreness (delayed onset muscle soreness, or DOMS) after exercise.

5. Improved Balance and Coordination: Warm-ups that include balance and coordination exercises can help reduce the risk of falls.

6. Increased Blood Flow: Warm-ups increase blood flow to the muscles, which helps deliver oxygen and nutrients.

7. Mental Preparation: Warm-ups can help mentally prepare seniors for physical activity, improving focus and concentration.

8. Reduced Risk of Chronic Conditions: Regular warm-ups can help manage chronic conditions like diabetes, hypertension, and heart disease.

9. Improved Functional Movement: Warm-ups that

include functional movements (like squats, lunges, and step-ups) can improve daily functioning and mobility.

10. Enhanced Overall Fitness: Warm-ups can improve overall fitness and well-being, enabling seniors to perform daily activities with more energy and confidence.

Remember, warm-ups should be gentle, gradual, and specific to the activity or exercise that follows. Consult with a healthcare professional or fitness expert to create a personalized warm-up routine.

Gentle Cardiovascular Warm-up Exercises

Here are some gentle cardiovascular warm-up exercises suitable for seniors over 60:

1. Brisk Walking: Walking quickly at a comfortable pace, about 3-4 miles per hour.

2. Marching in Place: Standing in one place, bringing knees up towards the chest, and marching.

3. Leg Swings: Standing with feet hip-width apart, swinging one leg forward and backward, then switching to the other leg.

4. Arm Circles: Holding arms straight out to the sides, making small circles with hands.

5. Seated Leg Lifts: Sitting in a chair, lifting one leg off the floor, and holding for a few seconds before lowering.

6. Wall Push-Ups: Standing with feet shoulder-width apart, hands on a wall at shoulder height, and slowly lowering body toward the wall.

7. Seated Arm Raises: Sitting in a chair, raising one arm straight out to the side, and holding for a few seconds before lowering.

8. Gentle Jogging in Place: Standing in one place, bringing knees up towards the chest, and jogging in place.

9. Side Steps: Standing with feet together, taking small steps to one side, and then the other.

10. Heel Taps: Standing with feet together, lifting one foot off the ground, and tapping the heel on the floor.

Remember to:

- Start slowly and gradually increase intensity and duration.

- Pay attention to your body's signals and take a break when necessary.

- Warm up for 5-10 minutes before exercise or physical activity.

- Consult with a healthcare professional or fitness expert to modify or add exercises based on individual needs and abilities.

Chapter 3

Strength Training for Seniors

Strength training, also known as resistance training, is a type of physical activity designed to improve muscular strength and endurance. It involves using resistance, such as weights, resistance bands, or one's body weight, to challenge muscles and stimulate growth and strength gains.

Strength training can be done with:

1. Free weights (dumbbells, barbells)

2. Resistance bands

3. Machines at the gym

4. Bodyweight exercises (push-ups, squats, lunges)

5. Resistance tubes

6. Kettlebells

7. Medicine balls

Strength training can be adapted to suit different fitness levels and goals, from beginner to advanced, and can be incorporated into a comprehensive fitness program to improve overall health and well-being.

Strength training is an essential component of fitness for seniors, helping to:

1. Build muscle mass and strength

2. Improve bone density

3. Improve stability and coordination

4. Increase mobility and flexibility

5. Support functional movements and daily activities

6. Reduce the risk of falls and injuries

7. Manage chronic conditions like diabetes, hypertension, and heart disease

8. Improve mental health and cognitive function

Some tips for strength training for seniors include:

1. Begin at a slow pace and advance steadily over time.

2. Focus on compound exercises like squats, lunges, and chest presses

3. Use lighter weights and higher repetitions (10-15 reps)

4. Incorporate bodyweight exercises like push-ups, squats, and lunges

5. Use resistance bands or machines at the gym

6. Work on functional movements like standing up from a chair, walking, and balance exercises

7. Incorporate core strengthening exercises like planks and bridges

8. Make it fun and social by exercising with a friend or group

Some examples of strength training exercises for seniors include:

1. Squats

2. Lunges

3. Chest Presses

4. Seated Row

5. Shoulder Press

6. Bicep Curls

7. Tricep Extensions

8. Leg Press

9. Calf Raises

10. Planks

Remember to consult with a healthcare professional or fitness expert to create a personalized strength training program that suits your needs and abilities.

Guidelines for Resistance Training

1. Frequency: At least 2 days a week to strengthen muscles, and 2 days a week for balance activities.

2. Duration: 30 minutes a day, 5 days a week, for moderate-intensity aerobic activity.

3. Intensity: Moderate-intensity aerobic activity (brisk walking, 5 or 6 on a 10-point scale) or vigorous-intensity activity (jogging, running, 7 or 8 on a 10-point scale).

Types of exercise:

- Multi-joint exercises: squats, deadlifts, chest presses, rows, lat pull downs, shoulder presses, plank.

- Single-joint exercises: leg curls, knee extensions, hip extensions, hip abductions, calf raises, bicep curls.

5. Progression: Increase weight, resistance, or reps as strength improves.

6. Precautions: Consult a doctor before starting a new exercise program, especially if you have medical conditions or concerns.

7. **Combination:** Combine resistance training with aerobic activity and balance exercises for overall fitness.

Additional guidelines for resistance training:

1. Start slowly: Begin with lighter weights and progress gradually to avoid injury or burnout.

2. Focus on functional movements: Emphasize exercises

that mimic daily activities, such as squats, lunges, and step-ups.

8. Use proper form: Ensure correct technique to avoid injury and maximize benefits.

9. Incorporate balance exercises: Include exercises that challenge balance and stability, such as single-leg squats and heel-to-toe walking.

10. Work on core strength: Incorporate exercises that target the core muscles, such as planks and bridges.

11. Make it social: Exercise with a friend or group to enhance motivation and enjoyment.

12. Monitor progress: Keep track of exercises, weights, and reps to monitor progress and adjust the program as needed.

13. Consult a professional: Work with a fitness professional or healthcare provider to develop a personalized exercise program.

Remember, the key is to start slowly, progress gradually, and focus on functional movements and balance exercises to improve overall fitness and reduce the risk of injury.

Upper Body Exercises

Here are some upper body exercises suitable for seniors:

1. Seated Row: Using a resistance band or light dumbbells, sit with your feet flat on the floor and pull the weight towards your chest.

2. Shoulder Rolls: Roll your shoulders forward and backward in a circular motion.

3. Arm Circles: Hold arms straight out to the sides and make small circles with your hands.

4. Chest Press: Using light dumbbells or a resistance band, press the weight forward, extending your arms.

5. Bicep Curls: Using light dumbbells, curl your arms up towards your shoulders.

6. Tricep Extensions: Using a resistance band or light dumbbells, extend your arm straight behind you.

7. Wall Push-Ups: Stand with feet shoulder-width apart and hands on a wall at shoulder height, slowly lowering your body toward the wall.

8. Seated Dumbbell Shoulder Press: Sit with your feet flat on the floor and press dumbbells straight up over your head.

9. Arm Raises: Hold arms straight out to the sides and raise them up and down.

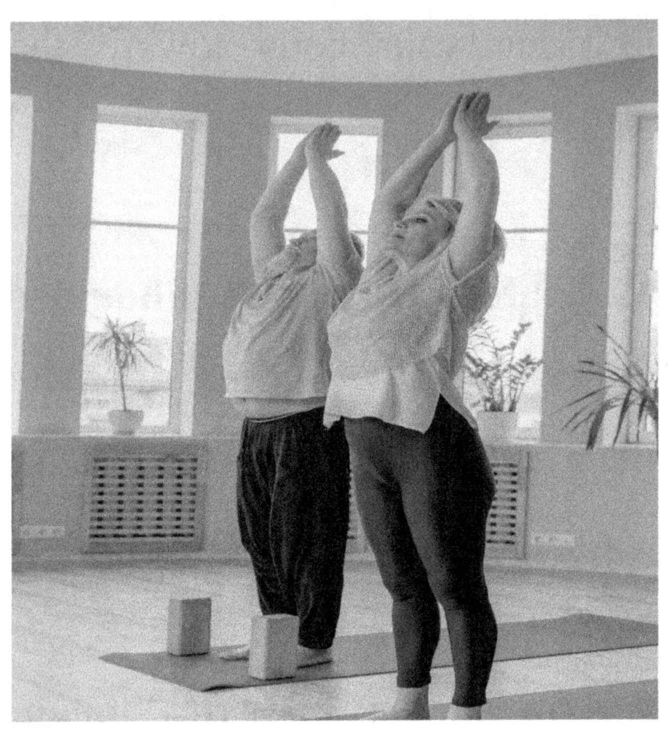

10. Resistance Band Chest Fly:

Hold a resistance band in both hands and press it outward, keeping your arms straight.

11. Seated Row with Rotation: Using a resistance band or light dumbbells, sit with your feet flat on the floor and pull the weight towards your chest, rotating your torso as you pull.

12. Shoulder Blade Squeeze: Sit or stand with good posture and squeeze your shoulder blades together.

13. Arm Across the Chest: Hold one arm straight out in front of you and bring the other arm across your body, holding your hand in place with your other hand.

14. Wall Angel: Stand with feet shoulder-width apart and hands on a wall at shoulder height, slowly lift your arms up and out to the sides, keeping your shoulders down and away from your ears.

15. Seated Dumbbell Lateral Raise: Sit with feet flat on the floor and hold dumbbells at your sides, lift the dumbbells out to the sides until they are at shoulder height.

Remember to:

Start slowly and gradually increase the number of repetitions and sets as you build strength and endurance.

- Focus on proper form and technique to avoid injury.

- Listen to your body and rest when needed.

- Consult with a healthcare professional or fitness expert to modify or add exercises based on individual needs and abilities.

It's also important to incorporate exercises that improve flexibility and range of motion, such as shoulder rolls and arm circles, to help maintain mobility and prevent stiffness in the upper body.

Lower Body Exercises

Here are some lower-body exercises suitable for seniors:

1. Seated Leg Lifts: Lift one leg off the floor, keeping the knee straight, and hold for a few seconds before lowering.

2. Seated Leg Press: Using a resistance band or light dumbbells, press one leg forward, extending your knee.

3. Seated Calf Raise: Lift your heels off the floor, raise your calves, and hold for a few seconds before lowering.

4. Standing Hip Flexion: Stand with feet shoulder-width apart and take a small step forward with one foot, keeping your knee straight.

5. Standing Hip Extension: Stand with feet shoulder-width apart and take a small step backward with one foot, keeping your knee straight.

6. Seated Knee Extension: Using a resistance band or light dumbbells, straighten your knee, lifting your foot off the floor.

7. Seated Ankle Rotation: Lift your feet off the floor and rotate your ankles in a circular motion.

8. Standing Toe Taps: Stand with feet together and lift one foot off the ground, tapping your toes on the floor in front of you.

9. Seated Heel Slides: Sit with your feet flat on the floor and slide your heels away from you, keeping your knees straight.

10. Standing Leg Raises: Stand with feet shoulder-width apart and lift one leg off the ground, holding for a few seconds before lowering.

Always remember to:

- Start slowly and gradually increase the number of repetitions and sets as you build strength and endurance.

- Focus on proper form and technique to avoid injury.

- Consult with a healthcare professional or fitness expert to modify or add exercises based on individual needs and abilities.

It's also important to incorporate exercises that improve balance and stability, such as single-leg squats and heel-to-toe walking, to help prevent falls and maintain mobility.

Core Exercises

1. Seated Marching: Sit with your feet flat on the floor and march in place, lifting your legs off the ground.

2. Seated Leg Circles: Lift your legs off the ground and make small circles with your feet.

3. Seated Hip Abductions: Lift your legs out to the sides, keeping them straight, and hold for a few seconds.

4. Seated Hip Adductions: Bring your legs together, keeping them straight, and hold for a few seconds.

5. Seated Torso Twist: Twist your torso from side to side, keeping your feet on the floor.

6. Seated Cat-Cow Stretch: Arch your back and lift your head and tailbone towards the ceiling (like a cat), then round your back and tuck your chin towards your chest (like a cow).

7. Seated Pelvic Clock: Imagine a clock on your pelvis and move your hips in a circular motion, first clockwise and then counterclockwise.

8. Seated Kegel Exercises: Contract and release your pelvic muscles, as if stopping the flow of urine.

9. Seated Bird Dog: Lift your arms and legs off the ground and hold for a few seconds, keeping your core muscles engaged.

10. Seated Side Plank: Lift your legs off the ground and balance on one side of your body, keeping your core muscles engaged.

11. Plank: Hold a plank position for 20-30 seconds, rest for 30 seconds, and repeat for 3-5 sets.

12. Seated Leg Raises: Lift your legs off the floor and hold for a few seconds, then lower them back down.

13. Seated Bicycle Crunches: Alternate bringing your knees towards your chest, as if pedaling a bicycle.

Remember to:

- Start slowly and gradually increase the number of repetitions and sets as you build strength and endurance.

- Focus on proper form and technique to avoid injury.

- Listen to your body and rest when needed.

- Consult with a healthcare professional or fitness expert

to modify or add exercises based on individual needs and abilities.

It's also important to incorporate exercises that challenge your balance and stability, such as single-leg squats and heel-to-toe walking, to help prevent falls and maintain mobility.

Chapter 4

Cardiovascular Exercises

Cardiovascular exercise, also known as cardio, is a type of physical activity that raises your heart rate and keeps it elevated for a sustained period. This type of exercise strengthens your heart and lungs, improving the body's ability to transport oxygen and nutrients to your cells.

Types of Cardiovascular Activities

1. Running or jogging

2. Swimming

3. Cycling

4. Brisk walking

5. Dancing

6. Aerobics classes

7. Jumping rope

8. Boxing or kickboxing

9. Rowing

10. High-intensity interval training (HIIT)

Regular cardiovascular exercise provides numerous health benefits, including:

- Improved heart health
- Increased lung function
- Enhanced circulation
- Weight management
- Reduced

Low-Impact Aerobic Exercises

1. Brisk Walking: Walking quickly at a pace of 3-4 miles per hour or faster.

2. Swimming or Water Aerobics: Gentle laps or water exercises that raise your heart rate.

3. Cycling or Stationary Bike: Gentle pedaling or using a stationary bike.

4. Tai Chi or Qigong: Gentle, slow movements that promote balance and cardiovascular health.

5. Chair Aerobics: Seated exercises that raise your heart rate, like arm raises and leg lifts.

6. Resistance Band Exercises: Gentle exercises using resistance bands to work your entire body.

7. Low-Impact Dance Classes: Gentle dance classes like line dancing or waltzing.

8. Seated Elliptical Trainer: A low-impact machine that simulates running without the impact.

9. Recumbent Bike: A bike that allows you to pedal with your legs while seated in a comfortable position.

10. Gentle Yoga or Pilates:

Modified exercises that focus on breathing, flexibility, and core strength.

Remember to:

- Start slowly and gradually increase intensity and duration.
- Listen to your body and rest when needed.

- Consult with a healthcare professional or fitness expert to modify or add exercises based on individual needs and abilities.

- Incorporate exercises that improve balance and flexibility to reduce the risk of falls.

These exercises are designed to be gentle on joints and muscles while still providing an effective cardiovascular workout. Always prioritize your safety and comfort.

Cardiovascular Workout Routine

Here is a sample cardiovascular workout routine:

Warm-up (5-10 minutes)

- Light cardio such as walking, jogging, or jumping jacks
- Dynamic stretching such as leg swings, arm circles, and hip rotations

Monday (30-45 minutes)

- Brisk walking, jogging, or running

- High-intensity interval training (HIIT) with sprints or hill climbs.

Wednesday (30-45 minutes)

- Swimming or water aerobics

Cycling or spinning

Thursday

Get a good rest

Friday (30-45 minutes)

- Dancing or Zumba
- Jumping rope or boxing/kickboxing

Sunday (30-45 minutes)

- Long, steady-state cardio such as jogging, cycling, or rowing
- Hill climbs or stair climbing.

Cool-down (5-10 minutes)

- Static stretching such as hamstring, quadriceps, and chest stretches

It's important to include rest days or active recovery days (e.g., light yoga or walking) to allow your body to recover and rebuild.

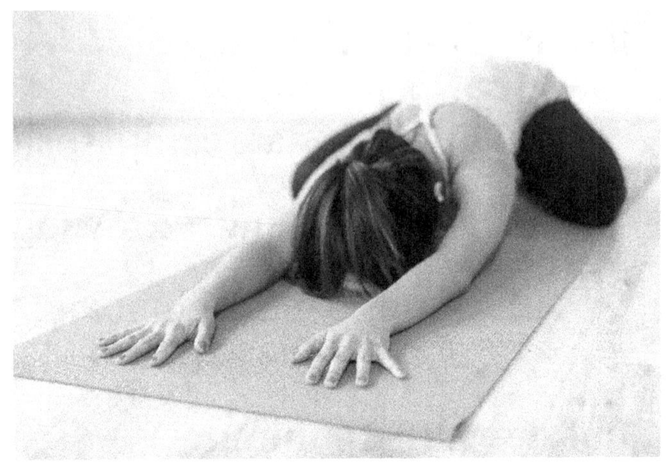

Chapter 5

Balance and Stability Exercises

1. Single-Leg Squats: Stand on one leg, bend your knee, and lower your body down, then stand back up.

2. Heel-To-Toe Walking with Eyes Closed: Walk along a straight line, placing the heel of one foot directly in front of the toes of the other foot, with your eyes closed.

3. Standing on a Soft Surface: Stand on a soft surface, like a mattress or a BOSU ball, to challenge your balance.

4. Balance Exercises with a Resistance Band: Use a resistance band to provide support and challenge your balance.

5. Seated Balance Exercises: Sit on a chair or bench and perform exercises like leaning forward and backward, side to side, and rotating your torso.

6. Standing with Feet Together:
Stand with your feet together, eyes closed, and hold for 30 seconds.

7. Walking in a Figure-Eight Pattern: Walk in a figure-eight pattern, crossing one foot over the other.

8. Standing on a Foam Pad with Eyes Closed: Stand on a foam pad, eyes closed, and hold for 30 seconds.

9. Balance Exercises with a Partner: Stand with a partner, hold hands, and perform exercises like leaning forward and backward, side to side, and rotating your torso.

10. Seated Marching: Sit on a chair or bench and lift your legs off the ground, marching in place.

11. Single-Leg Stance: Stand on one leg, holding onto a chair or wall for support.

12. Heel-To-Toe Walking: Walk along a straight line, placing the heel of one foot directly in front of the toes of the other foot.

13. Standing on Foam: Stand on a foam pad or cushion to challenge your balance.

14. Tai Chi or Qigong: Gentle, slow movements that promote balance and stability.

15. Standing Leg Lifts: Lift one leg off the ground, keeping it straight, and hold for a few seconds.

These exercises can help improve balance, reduce the risk of falls, and increase confidence in daily activities. Always prioritize safety and stability.

Importance of Balance and Stability

Balance and stability are crucial for seniors over 60 because:

1. Falls prevention: Good balance and stability can prevent falls, which are a leading cause of injury, disability, and death in older adults.

2. Mobility and independence: Balance and stability exercises help maintain mobility, enabling seniors to perform daily tasks and remain independent.

3. Reduced fear of falling: Improving balance and stability can reduce the fear of falling, which can limit activities and increase isolation.

4. Improved functional ability: Good balance and stability enable seniors to perform daily tasks, such as walking, standing, and changing direction.

5. Enhanced overall health: Balance and stability exercises can also improve overall health and well-being, reducing the risk of chronic diseases.

6. Cognitive function: Balance and stability exercises have been shown to improve cognitive function and reduce the risk of dementia.

7. Social engagement: Good balance and stability enable seniors to participate in social activities, reducing isolation and loneliness.

8. Reduced risk of injuries: Good balance and stability can prevent injuries from falls and other accidents.

9. Improved mental health:
Balance and stability exercises can reduce stress, anxiety, and depression.

10. Better quality of life:
Maintaining balance and stability can improve overall quality of life, enabling seniors to enjoy activities and live life to the fullest.

Remember, balance and stability are vital for seniors' overall health, mobility, and independence.

Regular exercises and practice can help maintain or improve them.

Exercises to Improve Balance

Here are some exercises to improve balance for seniors over 60:

1. Standing on One Foot: Stand on one foot, holding onto a chair or wall for support if needed.

2. Heel-To-Toe Walking: Walk along a straight line, placing the heel of one foot directly in front of the toes of the other foot.

3. Standing on a Foam Pad: Stand on a foam pad or cushion to challenge your balance.

4. Seated Leg Lifts: Lift one leg off the floor, keeping it straight, and hold for a few seconds.

5. Standing with Eyes Closed: Stand with your eyes closed, focusing on your balance.

6. Single-Leg Squats: Stand on one leg, bend your knee, and lower your body down, then stand back up.

7. Balance Exercises with a Walker: Use a walker to help with balance and stability.

8. Standing on a Soft Surface: Stand on a soft surface, like a mattress or BOSU ball, to challenge your balance.

9. Seated Balance Exercises: Sit on a chair or bench and perform exercises like leaning forward and

backward, side to side, and rotating your torso.

10. Walking in a Figure-Eight Pattern:

Walk in a figure-eight pattern, crossing one foot over the other.

Remember to:

- Start slowly and gradually increase difficulty
- Use support when needed
- Practice regularly to improve balance and stability

- Consult with a healthcare professional or fitness expert to modify or add exercises based on individual needs and abilities

These exercises can help improve balance, reduce the risk of falls, and increase confidence in daily activities.

Tai Chi and Yoga for Seniors

Tai Chi and Yoga are excellent exercises for seniors over 60, offering numerous benefits:

Tai Chi:

1. Improves balance and reduces fall risk

2. Enhances flexibility and mobility

3. Strengthens muscles and bones

4. Lowers blood pressure and improves cardiovascular health

5. Reduces stress and anxiety

6. Improves cognitive function and memory

7. Promotes relaxation and overall well-being

Yoga:

1. Increases flexibility and range of motion

2. Strengthens muscles and improves balance

3. Reduces stress and anxiety

4. Improves sleep quality

5. Enhances cardiovascular health

6. Supports bone health and reduces osteoporosis risk

7. Promotes relaxation and overall well-being

Modifications and considerations for seniors over 60

1. Start slowly and gradually increase intensity and duration

2. Use chairs, blocks, or straps for support and balance

3. Focus on gentle, low-impact movements

4. Avoid deep twists, bends, or complex poses

5. Practice breathing techniques and meditation for relaxation

6. Work with experienced instructors who specialize in senior fitness

7. Listen to your body and rest when needed

Remember to consult with your healthcare provider before starting any new exercise program. With gentle and mindful practice, Tai Chi and Yoga can be a wonderful way for seniors over 60 to improve their physical and mental well-being.

Chapter 6

Flexibility and Mobility Exercises

Flexibility and mobility exercises for seniors refer to activities that help maintain or improve the range of motion, flexibility, and mobility of joints, muscles, and other connective tissues.

Examples of flexibility and mobility exercises for seniors include:

1. Stretching exercises (e.g., neck stretches, shoulder rolls, hip flexor stretches)

2. Range of motion exercises (e.g., arm circles, leg swings, ankle rotations)

3. Mobility exercises (e.g., walking, marching, leg lifts)

4. Balance exercises (e.g., single-leg stance, heel-to-toe walking)

5. Gentle movements like tai chi, qigong, or yoga

6. Activities like swimming, cycling, or using an elliptical machine

7. Simple exercises like toe touches, knee bends, and leg stretches

Remember to:

- Start slowly and gradually increase intensity and duration
- Listen to your body and rest when needed
- Consult with a healthcare professional or fitness expert to create a personalized exercise plan

Incorporate exercises that work on strength, balance, and coordination for overall physical fitness.

Benefits of Flexibility and Mobility

Flexibility and mobility are crucial for seniors over 60, offering numerous benefits:

1. Improved daily functioning: Maintaining flexibility and mobility makes everyday activities easier, such as dressing, grooming, and bathing.

2. Reduced risk of falls: Flexibility and mobility exercises help improve balance and reduce the risk of falls and injuries.

3. Enhanced independence: Preserving flexibility and mobility enables seniors to maintain their independence and perform tasks without assistance.

4. Better overall health: Flexibility and mobility exercises can help manage chronic conditions like arthritis, diabetes, and heart disease.

5. Reduced pain: Improving flexibility and mobility can reduce joint pain and stiffness, improving overall comfort and quality of life.

6. Improved mental health: Exercise and physical activity can help reduce stress, anxiety, and depression in seniors.

7. Enhanced social engagement: Participating in flexibility and mobility exercises can provide opportunities for social interaction and community engagement.

8. Better sleep: Regular exercise, including flexibility and mobility exercises, can improve sleep quality and duration.

9. Increased energy: Improving flexibility and mobility can boost energy levels and reduce fatigue.

10. Extended mobility and independence: Preserving

flexibility and mobility can delay the need for assistive devices like canes, walkers, or wheelchairs.

Remember, it's never too late to start. Even small improvements in flexibility and mobility can make a significant difference in a senior's quality of life.

Yoga Poses for Flexibility

Here are some gentle and modified yoga poses that can help improve flexibility for seniors over 60:

1. Seated Forward Fold (Modified): Sit with legs straight out, lean forward, and reach for toes or shins.

2. Neck Stretch (Slow and Gentle): Slowly tilt head to the side, bringing ear towards shoulder.

3. Shoulder Rolls (Forward and Backward): Roll shoulders forward and backward in a circular motion.

4. Chest Expansion (Modified):

Stand in a doorway with arms up and hands on the doorframe, leaning forward slightly.

5. Hip Flexor Stretch (Modified):

Stand with one hand against a wall, take a large step forward with one foot, and bend the front knee.

6. Calf Stretch (Modified): Stand

facing a wall with one hand on the wall, step one foot back about a foot, and bend the front knee.

7. Seated Leg Stretch (Modified): Sit with legs straight out, lift one leg out to the side, and hold onto a strap or towel if needed.

8. Cat-Cow Stretch (Modified): Start on hands and knees, arch back, and lift your tailbone (like a cat), then round back and tuck chin to chest (like a cow).

9. Seated Twist (Modified): Sit with your legs crossed, twist your torso to one side, and hold onto a strap or towel if needed.

10. Leg Raises (Modified): Lie on your back, lift one leg a few inches off the ground, and hold for a few seconds before lowering.

Remember to:

- Start slowly and gently
- Listen to your body and rest when needed
- Use props or modifications to make poses more accessible
- Consult with a healthcare professional or yoga expert to create a personalized practice

These poses can help improve flexibility, balance, and overall mobility, but always prioritize safety and comfort.

Chapter 7

Managing Joint Pain and Arthritis

Managing joint pain and arthritis for seniors over 60 requires a comprehensive approach. Here are some strategies to help alleviate symptoms and improve quality of life:

1. Medications: Consult with your doctor about pain-relieving medications, such as acetaminophen or nonsteroidal anti-inflammatory drugs (NSAIDs).

2. Physical Therapy: Gentle exercises and physical therapy can help maintain joint mobility and strength.

3. Lifestyle Changes:

- Maintain a healthy weight to reduce pressure on joints.
- Engage in low-impact activities like walking, swimming, or cycling.

- Use assistive devices like canes or walkers if needed.

4. Alternative Therapies:

- Acupuncture
- Massage therapy
- Heat or cold therapy
- Yoga or tai chi (modified for seniors)

5. Assistive Devices:

- Joint braces or supports
- Orthotics or shoe inserts
- Adaptive equipment for daily activities

6. Surgery (if necessary): Consult with an orthopedic specialist about joint replacement or other surgical options.

7. Self-Management Techniques:

- Practice relaxation techniques like deep breathing or meditation

- Engage in activities that bring joy and help distract from pain

- Stay connected with friends and family for emotional support

8. Regular Medical Check-Ups:

Monitor your condition and adjust treatments as needed.

Remember to consult with your healthcare provider before starting any new therapies or treatments. By combining these approaches, seniors can effectively manage joint pain and arthritis, improving their overall well-being.

Tips for Dealing with Joint Pain

Here are some tips for dealing with joint pain for seniors over 60:

1. Stay Active: Gentle exercises like walking, swimming, or yoga can help reduce stiffness and improve joint mobility.

2. Maintain a Healthy Weight: Excess weight puts additional strain on joints, so managing weight through diet and exercise can help alleviate pain.

3. Use Assistive Devices: Canes, walkers, or orthotics can help reduce pressure on joints and improve mobility.

4. Practice Good Posture: Maintaining proper posture can reduce strain on joints and alleviate pain.

5. Take Breaks: Rest and ice joints regularly to reduce inflammation and pain.

6. Stay Hydrated: Drinking plenty of water helps keep joints lubricated and healthy.

7. Manage Stress: Stress can exacerbate pain; engage in relaxation techniques like meditation or deep breathing.

8. Get Enough Sleep: Adequate sleep helps reduce pain and inflammation.

9. Try Heat or Cold Therapy: Applying heat or cold packs can help reduce pain and stiffness.

10. Consider Physical Therapy: A physical therapist can help develop a personalized exercise program to improve joint mobility and strength.

11. Stay Connected: Social support from friends, family, or support groups can help cope with pain and improve mental well-being.

12. Consult a Healthcare Professional: Regular check-ups with your doctor or orthopedic specialist can help manage pain and address any underlying conditions.

Exercises to Alleviate Arthritis Symptoms

Here are some exercises that can help alleviate arthritis symptoms for seniors over 60:

1. Range of Motion Exercises: Gentle movements to maintain joint mobility, such as arm circles, leg swings, and hip rotations.

2. Strengthening Exercises: Building muscle around affected joints, like leg lifts, arm raises, and shoulder presses.

3. Low-Impact Aerobics: Activities like walking, swimming, cycling, or tai chi to improve cardiovascular health without excessive joint stress.

4. Flexibility Exercises: Gentle stretching to maintain flexibility, such as hamstring, hip flexor, and shoulder stretches.

5. Balance and Coordination Exercises: Activities like single-leg standing, heel-to-toe walking, or tai chi to improve balance and reduce fall risk.

6. Water-Based Exercises: Aquatic exercises or water aerobics to reduce joint stress while improving mobility and strength.

7. Resistance Band Exercises: Using resistance bands to strengthen muscles without excessive joint strain.

8. Gentle Yoga or Pilates: Modified exercises to improve flexibility, balance, and strength while minimizing joint impact.

9. Breathing and Relaxation Exercises: Techniques like deep breathing, meditation, or progressive muscle relaxation to manage pain and reduce stress.

10. Functional Activities: Exercises that mimic daily activities, like squats, lunges, or step-ups, to improve mobility and strength for everyday tasks.

Remember to:

- Consult with your healthcare provider or physical therapist before starting new exercises

- Start slowly and gradually increase intensity and duration

- Listen to your body and rest when needed

- Use proper technique and form to avoid injury

These exercises can help alleviate arthritis symptoms, improve mobility, and enhance the overall quality of life for seniors over 60.

Chapter 8

Exercise Modifications and Adaptations

Exercise modifications and adaptations are essential for seniors over 60, especially those with arthritis or other mobility limitations. Here are some tips to modify exercises and make them more accessible:

1. Start slow and gradually increase intensity and duration.

2. Use chairs, walls, or other support for balance and stability.

3. Replace high-impact exercises with low-impact alternatives (e.g., swimming or cycling instead of running).

4. Use resistance bands or light weights instead of heavy weights.

5. Shorten the range of motion or reduce the depth of movements.

6. Take regular breaks to rest and stretch.

7. Use assistive devices like canes or walkers for support.

8. Modify exercises to avoid putting excessive strain on joints (e.g., avoid deep squats or lunges).

9. Use pool exercises or water-based activities for low-impact, gentle movements.

10. Work with a physical therapist or fitness professional to create a personalized exercise plan.

Some examples of modified exercises include:

- Seated leg lifts instead of squats

- Wall push-ups instead of traditional push-ups
- Seated arm raises instead of overhead presses
- Chair yoga or tai chi instead of traditional yoga or tai chi
- Using a stationary bike instead of a treadmill

Remember, it's essential to prioritize safety and comfort when exercising, especially for seniors with mobility limitations. Always consult with a healthcare professional or fitness expert to create a personalized exercise plan.

Customizing Workouts for Individual Needs

Customizing workouts for individual needs is crucial, especially for seniors over 60. Here are some factors to consider when tailoring a workout plan:

1. **Health status:** Consider any health conditions, such as arthritis, diabetes, or heart disease, and modify exercises accordingly.

2. Fitness level: Start with gentle exercises and gradually increase intensity and duration as fitness improves.

3. Mobility and flexibility: Adapt exercises to accommodate mobility limitations or flexibility issues.

4. Goals: Set specific goals, such as improving balance, increasing strength, or enhancing cardiovascular health.

5. Preferences: Incorporate exercises that are enjoyable and engaging to promote consistency.

6. Age and abilities: Consider age-related changes and physical abilities when selecting exercises.

7. Medical clearance: Obtain medical clearance before starting a new exercise program, especially if you have underlying health conditions.

8.   Progressive   overload: Gradually increase exercise intensity and difficulty as fitness improves.

9. Balance and coordination: Incorporate exercises that challenge balance and coordination to reduce fall risk.

10. Social support: Exercise with a partner or group for motivation and social interaction.

Some examples of customized workouts include:

- Chair yoga for mobility and flexibility

- Water aerobics for cardiovascular health and joint support

- Resistance band exercises for strength training

- Balance exercises like single-leg squats or heel-to-toe walking

- Gentle stretching for flexibility and range of motion

Remember to consult with a healthcare professional or fitness expert to create a personalized workout plan that suits your unique needs and goals.

Exercises for Seniors with Limited Mobility

Exercises for seniors with limited mobility can be modified to accommodate physical limitations and improve overall health. Here are some examples:

1. Seated exercises

1. Chair squats

2. Seated leg lifts

3. Arm raises

4. Shoulder rolls

5. Chest presses

2. Bed exercises

- Leg lifts

- Arm circles

- Shoulder rolls

- Chest presses

- Deep breathing exercises

3. Gentle stretching

- Neck stretches

- Shoulder stretches

- Chest stretches

- Hip flexor stretches

- Calf stretches

4. Resistance band exercises

- Arm curls

- Leg curls

- Chest presses

- Shoulder rotations

5. Breathing exercises

- Deep breathing

- Diaphragmatic breathing

- Box breathing

6. Range of motion exercises

- Shoulder rotations

- Elbow extensions

- Wrist extensions

- Hip rotations

- Knee extensions

7. Balance exercises

- Seated balance exercises

- Standing balance exercises (with support)

8. Mental stimulation

- Memory games

- Word puzzles

- Card games

- Reading

Remember to:

- Consult with a healthcare professional or physical therapist before starting any new exercise program

- Start slowly and gradually increase intensity and duration

- Listen to your body and rest when needed
- Use proper technique and form to avoid injury

These exercises can help improve flexibility, strength, balance, and overall well-being for seniors with limited mobility.

Adapting Workouts for Those with Chronic Conditions

Adapting workouts for individuals with chronic conditions requires careful consideration of their specific needs and limitations. Here are some tips to adapt workouts for common chronic conditions:

1. Arthritis:

- Gentle, low-impact exercises like yoga, swimming, or cycling
- Avoid high-impact activities like running or jumping
- Use resistance bands or light weights for strength training

2. Diabetes:

- Regular aerobic exercise like brisk walking, cycling, or swimming

- Incorporate strength training to improve insulin sensitivity

- Monitor blood sugar levels before and after exercise

3. Heart Disease:

- Cardiac rehabilitation programs or supervised exercise programs

- Aerobic exercises like walking, swimming, or cycling

- Avoid high-intensity exercises or those that increase blood pressure

4. Chronic Obstructive Pulmonary Disease (COPD):

- Breathing exercises and pulmonary rehabilitation programs
- Gentle aerobic exercises like walking or swimming
- Avoid exercises that exacerbate symptoms or trigger shortness of breath

5. Fibromyalgia:

- Gentle, low-impact exercises like yoga, tai chi, or swimming

- Avoid high-impact activities or those that cause pain

- Incorporate stress-reducing techniques like meditation or deep breathing

6. Osteoporosis:

- Weight-bearing exercises like walking, jogging, or weightlifting

- Incorporate balance and fall prevention exercises

- Avoid high-impact activities or those that increase the risk of fracture

7. Stroke or Neurological Conditions:

- Physical therapy or rehabilitation programs
- Gentle exercises like walking, swimming, or cycling
- Incorporate cognitive and memory exercises

Remember to:

- Consult with a healthcare professional or fitness expert

to create a personalized exercise plan

- Start slowly and gradually increase intensity and duration

- Listen to your body and rest when needed

- Use proper technique and form to avoid injury

By adapting workouts to individual needs and limitations, individuals with chronic conditions can safely and effectively improve their physical fitness and overall health.

Chapter 9

Staying Motivated and Creating a Workout Routine

Staying motivated and creating a workout routine can be challenging, but here are some tips to help:

1. Set specific and achievable goals

2. Find an exercise you enjoy

3. Vary your routine to avoid boredom

4. Schedule workouts in your calendar

5. Find a workout buddy or accountability partner

6. Track progress through a journal or app

7. Reward yourself for milestones reached

8. Make it convenient (find a gym close to home or work)

9. Focus on how you feel, not just physical appearance

10. Be kind to yourself and don't give up.

Creating a workout routine:

1. Start with a consultation with a fitness professional

2. Assess your fitness level and goals

3. Create a balanced routine (cardio, strength training, flexibility)

4. Include warm-ups and cool-downs

5. Start slowly and gradually increase intensity and duration

6. Make it realistic and sustainable

7. Include rest days and active recovery

8. Monitor progress and adjust when needed.

Setting Realistic Goals

Setting realistic goals is crucial for achieving success and maintaining motivation. Here are some tips for setting realistic goals:

1. Make your goals specific, measurable, achievable, relevant, and time-bound (SMART).

2. Set short-term and long-term goals.

3. Break down large goals into smaller, manageable tasks.

4. Consider your current fitness level and abilities.

5. Set goals that are challenging but not impossible.

6. Make sure your goals align with your values and priorities.

7. Write down your goals and track progress.

8. Be flexible and willing to adjust your goals as needed.

9. Celebrate your successes along the way.

10. Get support from a friend, family member, or fitness professional.

Examples of realistic goals:

- "I want to walk for 30 minutes, 3 times a week, for the next 3 months to improve my cardiovascular health."
- "I aim to do 3 sets of 10 reps of squats, 2 times a week, for the next 6 weeks to strengthen my legs."
- "I want to reduce my body fat percentage from 30% to 25%

in the next 6 months by eating a balanced diet and exercising regularly."

Remember, setting realistic goals is about making progress, not perfection. It's about setting yourself up for success and enjoying the journey towards a healthier and happier you.

Finding Workout Buddies

Finding workout buddies can be a great way to stay motivated and accountable. Here are some ways to find a workout buddy:

1. Ask friends or family members to join you

2. Join a fitness class or group training program

3. Use social media to find workout buddies in your area

4. Post on local community boards or apps

5. Join a running or cycling club

6. Participate in fitness events or challenges

7. Ask a personal trainer for guidance

8. Use online platforms or apps that connect workout buddies

9. Invite coworkers or colleagues to join you

10. Join a recreational sports team or league

Benefits of having a workout buddy:

1. Accountability

2. Motivation

3. Social support

4. Variety in workouts

5. Safety

6. Fun and enjoyment

7. Shared experience and camaraderie

8. Healthy competition

9. Learning new exercises and techniques

10. Celebrating progress and successes together.

Workout Routine For Seniors Over 60

Monday (Upper Body and Balance)

1. Warm-up: 5-minute walk or light cardio

2. Seated arm raises (3 sets of 10 reps)

3. Seated shoulder press (3 sets of 10 reps)

4. Wall push-ups (3 sets of 10 reps)

5. Single-leg stance (3 sets of 30 seconds per leg)

6. Cool-down: 5-minute stretching

Tuesday (Lower Body and Flexibility)

1. Warm-up: 5-minute walk or light cardio

2. Seated leg lifts (3 sets of 10 reps)

3. Calf raises (3 sets of 15 reps)

4. Seated leg stretches (3 sets of 30 seconds per leg)

5. Hip flexor stretches (3 sets of 30 seconds per leg)

6. Cool-down: 5-minute stretching

Wednesday (Rest day)

Get a good rest , to remove strains.

Thursday (Core and Balance)

1. Warm-up: 5-minute walk or light cardio

2. Seated bicycle crunches (3 sets of 10 reps)

3. Seated Russian twists (3 sets of 10 reps)

4. Single-leg stance with eyes closed (3 sets of 30 seconds per leg)

5. Heel-to-toe walking (3 sets of 10 steps)

6. Cool-down: 5-minute stretching

Friday (Upper Body and Cardio)

1. Warm-up: 5-minute walk or light cardio

2. Seated rowing exercises (3 sets of 10 reps)

3. Seated bicep curls (3 sets of 10 reps)

4. Brisk walking (3 sets of 5 minutes)

5. Cool-down: 5-minute stretching

Saturday and Sunday (Rest days)

Remember To:

- Start with lighter weights and progress gradually

- Rest for 30-60 seconds between sets

- Focus on proper form and technique

- Consult with a healthcare professional or fitness expert to modify the routine as needed

Remember to listen to your body and rest when needed. It's also essential to incorporate activities you enjoy, such as swimming, dancing, or gardening, to keep your workouts fun and engaging.

Chapter 10

Frequently Asked Questions (FAQs)

Here are some frequently asked questions (FAQs) about senior over 60 workouts:

Q: What is the best exercise for seniors over 60?

A: The best exercises for seniors over 60 are low-impact, gentle, and progressive, such as brisk walking, swimming, yoga, tai chi, and weight training.

Q: How often should seniors over 60 exercise?

A: Seniors over 60 should aim to exercise at least 3-4 times per week, with at least one day of rest in between.

Q: What are the benefits of exercise for seniors over 60?

A: Exercise can help seniors over 60 improve flexibility, balance, strength, and cardiovascular health, and reduce the risk of chronic diseases like diabetes, heart disease, and some cancers.

Q: Can seniors over 60 start a new exercise routine?

A: Yes, seniors over 60 can start a new exercise routine, but it's essential to consult with a healthcare professional or fitness expert to create a personalized and safe plan.

Q: How long should seniors over 60 exercise each session?

A: Exercise sessions for seniors over 60 should last around 30-45 minutes, including warm-up and cool-down periods.

Q: What are some exercises that seniors over 60 should avoid?

A: Seniors over 60 should avoid high-impact exercises like running, jumping, and heavy weightlifting, as well as exercises that involve bending or twisting.

Q: Can seniors over 60 exercise with chronic conditions like arthritis or diabetes?

A: Yes, seniors over 60 with chronic conditions can exercise, but they should consult with their healthcare provider to create a modified exercise plan that takes into account their condition and any limitations.

Q: How can seniors over 60 stay motivated to exercise?

A: Seniors over 60 can stay motivated to exercise by finding an exercise buddy, setting achievable goals, tracking progress, and rewarding themselves for milestones reached.

What Should Seniors Eat to Support Their Fitness Journey?

1. Eat a balanced diet: Seniors should eat a variety of foods from each food group to meet daily nutritional needs. Choose foods with little to no added sugar, saturated fats, and sodium.

2. Add more fiber: Fiber reduces constipation, helps with weight loss, reduces the risk of diabetes, pre-diabetes, heart disease, and colon cancer, and lowers blood cholesterol levels. Men over 50 should get 30 grams of fiber per day; women over 50 should get 21 grams per day. Good sources of fiber include beans, whole grains, vegetables, and fruits.

3. Eat more protein: Seniors should consume about one gram of protein per kilogram (2.2 pounds) of body weight to prevent muscle loss. Good sources of protein include wild salmon, whole eggs, organic whey protein powder, and grass-fed beef.

4. Drink plenty of water: Seniors should drink 64 ounces of water per day, and can also get part of it from foods that are naturally rich in water, such as cucumbers and tomatoes.

5. Eat small, frequent meals: Eating small meals and snacks throughout the day can help keep your metabolism going. Aim not to go more than 3 hours without eating.

6. Avoid processed foods and drinks: Processed foods contain sugars, saturated fats, and other harmful additives. Instead, choose healthier foods like vegetables, eggs, and whole grains.

7. Reduce sugar intake: Consuming refined sugar has been linked to health conditions like diabetes and high blood pressure. Swap sugary treats with nutritious alternatives.

8. Stay hydrated: Water is vital for a balanced diet. Staying hydrated can boost metabolism, aid digestion, and reduce joint pain.

Conclusion

Encouragement for Seniors to Make

1. You are never too old to start making positive changes in your life.

2. Every small step counts, and it's okay to start slow.

3. Your health and well-being are worth the effort.

4. You've got this. You've overcome challenges before, and you can do it again.

5. Remember, it's not about adding years to your life, but about adding life to your years.

6. You're an inspiration to others, and your healthy habits will have a positive impact on those around you.

7. It's never too late to take control of your health and fitness.

8. You're capable of more than you think, and you'll be amazed at what you can accomplish.

9. Don't be afraid to ask for help or support - you don't have to do it alone.

10. Celebrate your small victories along the way - they add up and will keep you motivated.

Bonus videos

Scan the QR code to redirect to videos